The Art Of

Selling

Personal

Training

Mike Bell

The Art Of Selling Personal Training

Copyright © 2018 by Mike Bell

Printed in USA

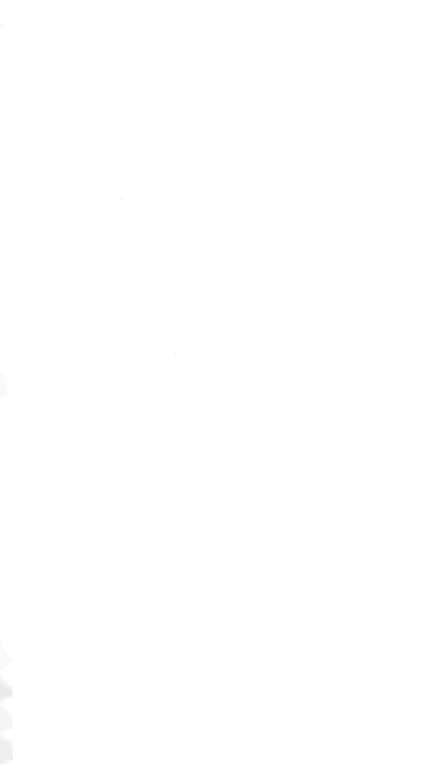

Table of Contents

Introduction   6

The Formula   12

4 Things Needed To Make A Sale   24

5 Step Sales Process   32

Diagrams   43

Workout   55

Price Presentation   60

Overcoming Objections   67

Bonus Material   98

Introduction

I had just heard that dreaded phrase from my boss, "Mike we need to have a talk." I knew it wasn't going to be good. I had been with the company for 2 months now but still hadn't made one personal training sale. I loved my job and loved helping people but for some reason I couldn't close anyone.

What made this even more weird to me was that I came from AT&T where I was constantly in the top 10% of 26,000 employees in sales. I've won tons of awards and was very successful. So when I left them to join the fitness industry I was in for a total shock when 2 months into my career I was sitting across from the district manager who is absolutely infuriated with my performance.

I didn't understand it. Every single person I sat with LOVED my session with them. They couldn't wait to work out again and many of them had joyful tears after our session together. Yet when it came to buying personal training all of them would say to me, "Mike I loved everything I just really need to think it over. Can I get back with you tomorrow?" Anxiously I would wait the next day and make that awkward phone call just to find out they weren't able to do it.

I had worked out over 100 people before my district manager came storming into my club to have a word with me. Maybe he didn't believe I was working, but after I showed him over $40,000 worth of potential sales sitting on my desk with name after name of person interested in changing their lives, he realized I was actually very hard at work.

I learned a strong lesson those first two months and it was this-
1) Personality, great work outs, and charisma are not enough to sell personal training. This was something totally different than selling a car or up-selling people to buy a tablet with their phone or a home security system. What this needed was a process and without the process it was near impossible to close a sale.

2) I quickly learned that 98% of people who left my desk weren't ever coming back. You're either selling them on wanting to change their life or they are selling you on an excuse. Someone is

surely selling someone, the question is who.

After meeting with my district manager, I sat looking at the $40,000 in personal training sales I could have made and was so frustrated. I tried over and over to close people but just couldn't close anyone. It was in that moment that I made a decision few people would make. I grabbed all those manuals of potential sales and tore them into pieces and decided from then on that if someone left my desk, there's a great chance they are never coming back. I needed to get good, actually not just good but exceptional if I was going to be able to keep my job and further my career.

After applying the principles I learned in this book, I was able to sell more than

$540,000 in personal training sales my first year with the company. I quickly moved up from sales counselor to assistant manager and within a matter of months was running one of the most successful personal training gyms the company had ever seen which averaged $70,000 a month in reoccurring revenues. I had grown the EFT base from $40,000 a month to $70,000 a month my first year. Within that same year I was then promoted at the age of 28 to District Vice President and began teaching the structure that taught me how to be successful to all the other managers in the district. I know this may sound absurd to you and may not sound possible, but listen to every single word I say. I'll prove this system over and over.

Through this book you'll learn a lot. But I can't stress enough the importance of memorizing the scripts I'm going to provide for you. It's not personality that sells….. it's the process. I can take any person off the streets and show them this process and if they follow it PERFECTLY they WILL make a SALE. Fail to follow it perfectly and you will massively struggle in your sales efforts.

The Formula

Before I was promoted to District Vice President, I constantly battled in sales with one of my best friends who worked at a different location. He was a giant guy whose body was as big as his heart! Everyone loved him and he was very successful in his career at selling personal training. Month after month he would sell about 15-25k in personal training sales. Yet month after month I was around 40-50k in sales.

One day when I was finally promoted up to District Vice President I visited his club and asked him this question-

Moose, are you outgoing?

He's like, "Of course!"

Do people usually like you?

"Yea Mike"

And you have a solid work out correct?

"Mike you know how awesome it is."

Then Moose, how come my sales were always twice the amount of yours?

He sat down and thought for a second and responded, "I don't know."

So I proceeded to say, "Moose I truly believe that you and I are almost the exact same person as far as personality goes and style goes. The only reason I feel why my sales are twice yours is because my presentation is different than yours…would you agree?"

And surely my presentation was different than his. He was a hard angle closer as people liked to refer to him. He liked pushing people into the corner and making them decide today. He would cause that sweating on their foreheads as they stumbled with words trying to push away his techniques but simply not finding a way. He would use phrases like, "If I could…..would you?" and "What could possibly be stopping you from starting with me today?" Which would often cause them to feel heavily pressured. I on the other hand take quite the opposite approach. I don't want people to feel pressured nor like I'm selling them. I want them to feel like they are talking to a friend and that I am there to help them.

This whole program is to create those feelings in your members. But the only way you can keep from becoming a pushy salesman is by learning what I like to call THE FORMULA.

The foundational aspect that must be memorized if you are to ever see a significant shift in your personal training sales is understanding this formula-

Verbals+NonVerbals

$---$ Create $--> \quad$ 1) feelings

$$---$$

2) Response

Everything you say and do produces two things in a person- a feeling and a response.
If you don't like their response (aka: no thank you, not right now, can I think about it, I'm not sure) , change their feelings. To change their feelings you

must change your verbals or non verbals. It's that simple.

Let me give you an example: If I say to someone, "Would you like a free personal training session?" Most people will actually say, "No I'm not interested." or "No, not right now." Very few will actually say, "Great!"

Why would most people deny a free session? It's because of the formula. It's not what you say but how you say what you say. Your words are creating a feeling in that person, and they are most likely feeling like there's a catch to that free session. Maybe they feel like you are just trying to sell them personal training instead of just helping them; which is why most people will pass on the free session. Now let's change your words to, "Hey Mary, for member appreciation day your account was given a free training session. When are you coming to the gym next?"

Surprisingly she will be excited and give you a date and time.

The reason she gives you an answer is because she FEELS like she won something and isn't being sold something. And therefore her response is to give you a date and time for a session.

You are in direct control of how people respond to you as an individual. If you don't like the responses you have been getting, it's because of the feelings you gave them which came from what you said or from your non verbals.

If someone felt like they were being sold by a car salesman...you created that feeling....with your words and how you approached that sales process.

If they were excited about your work out.....you created that feeling.
If they keep saying that they need to talk to their spouse or think about it....you lead them to that response.

The formula is simple...if you don't like the responses you are getting from people, then change what you say and how you say it.
I've learned that every single person in front of me is like a white piece of paper and with the words I use I have the ability to paint a beautiful picture of emotional bliss or with a different choice of words to paint the darkest photos that push people away. We're either leading people toward the water to take a drink, pushing them away, or just not able to lead them at all. And the only way any of those 3 aspects are done is through your words.

CONVERSATION CONTROL

So if its true that there is a formula with how our communication is processed in an individual, that also means that if given a certain sequence of words we should be able to predict the answer before we get it. This is what is called conversation control. In other words, when engaging with someone I am going to ask a series of questions that I already know the answers to so that I can lead the person to what I am trying to do. An important thing to understand psychologically in this process is this- I am making them feel like they are the ones in control because I am asking questions instead of telling them what to do which gives them a feeling of choice even though I am really not giving them an option.

For example-

If someone says to me at the end of a personal training sale that they need to think about it… I respond back with-

"Did you want to think about getting in shape or was it more about the money?"

You see I am giving them two choices which makes them feel in control and I am leading the conversation to where I want it; to talk about the money and find a program that actually fits the budget.

The wrong approach is to push someone away with your words by saying things like, "Think about it? What's their to think about? You're 40% body fat and haven been able to get to your goal in over 2 years. I seriously don't understand what you need to think about. You need to get started before something worse happens."

As you can see from those sentences, you are causing emotions of defense in the person and pushing them away.

Some of you might say to me, "Mike I would never say anything like that."

Well I've heard many people say those exact kind of things and we need to stay clear of it. The most common human response to an objection is to prove that person wrong and begin an argument. You will never make a sale by getting into an argument. Instead you need to learn to redirect the conversation by the use of questions through conversation control. Sounds hard, but its really just learning to dissect how a sentence is structured so that it yields the best response. The simplest way is forming your sentence to the FEEL, FELT, FOUND sentence structure. In essence, you always want to handle objections with a feel, felt, found sentence structure (I understand how you feel, in fact many people have felt that same way, but what many have come to find out is…); I will explain more on this later.

When I open my mouth I am aware of multiple things happening at once:
1) How open is the person to me right now (Do they like me yet? Are they engaging?)
2) What is this person feeling right now (Do they look confused? Are they happy? Are they feeling excited? Do they feel like I'm just trying to take from them?)

From there you can know whether you need to pull back or move in.

So we use the Formula and Conversation Control in each of the 5 steps in the sales process that I will explain below in order to lead a person toward buying personal training. If you are giving away free session with not actual process, selling personal training is going to be very difficult. In fact, if you follow the process I am going to give you, you don't even need to give multiple workouts. One will be good enough.

Remember, the whole basis of everything I am about to explain hinges on this formula and using conversation control. It is impossible to get really good at sales by just guessing. You need to know what you're doing, why you are doing it, and how to lead that person to a sale without making them feel like they are being sold.

4 Things Needed To Make A Sale

There are 4 things needed to make a sale….if these are not in your presentation, then this is why you are missing sales.

1) Need

It seems stupid to say this, but so many trainers I work with fail to realize that they didn't make the person FEEL like they NEED a trainer. Ninety percent of people don't buy training because they think they can do it on their own. I mean think of it, someone joins the gym because they really believe that they know what to do to get in shape. Therefore, why pay thousands of dollars if they can do it themselves? The problem is that it's your job through the presentation to show them that they don't know that they don't know how to reach their goals. Everyone joins the gym with the same presumption- "all I need to do to lose weight is go to the gym, run a little bit and hit a few machines." They just don't realize that unfortunately that plan doesn't work and that's why seventy percent of people quit the gym after 3 months of joining. It's your job to get them to say that they need you. Key words- get THEM TO SAY they need you...not you telling them. Surely you can tell someone that they need training and may feel deep down inside that they need training, but unless they actually say it aloud to you with their own mouth, they will likely not buy from you.

The reality is that if someone doesn't need you, or feel they need you, then why would they buy from you? Again, it's your job to show them they need you. How do you do this? By following the sales process I'm going to teach you in the next chapter.

2) Emotions

What I mean by emotions is how motivated is the person in front of you willing to change their lives? People change for one of two reasons as Tony Robbins explains, "Inspiration or desperation." Either they are sitting in front of you because they have been inspired by someone or they are sitting in front of you because they have no other choice but to change their life. Now wouldn't you agree that each person you sit in front of is at a different scale of how badly they want it? Sure, everyone says they want to get in shape and most people say they are really motivated, but you must not be fooled by their words. If someone says on a scale of 1-10 that they are an 8 as far as motivated…then I will tell you right now that they are not motivated enough to buy training.

You must know that it is your job get each person at a 10. If they are not at a 10 emotionally, it is going to be really hard to get them to buy today because they will want to just think about it. People who want to change their lives don't "Think about it". You must get them to a spot emotionally where they are absolutely certain that today is the day that they are going to change their lives forever. I will teach you how to do this with your words through conversation control and the formula so you can easily get people to do this. Psychologically this is called pre-framing the person. And another technique to get people emotionally invested is by challenging their own statements which I will show you. For instance, when someone says they are going to change their life this next year I will challenge them and say, "Are you sure you're really ready for this kind of commitment?"

They will be more intense at saying, "Yes."

I will follow up one more time with, "So you're not going to back out on me or quit or make excuses like everyone else does?"

As you can see, through my sentence choices I am getting this person more and more emotionally committed to changing their life.

Then after all of that I will tie them down with their own words, "So it sounds like to me that you are extremely serious about getting in the best shape of your life…is that correct?"

3) Value

Either they believe that what you are offering is going to get them to their goals or it's not. If the person doesn't believe you can get them to their goals then obviously they don't see the value in spending $200 a month in personal training and therefore aren't going to buy it.

4) Urgency

Why should they buy today when they can buy tomorrow? Unless you can create a compelling reason on why today is better than any other day then you will constantly fall into the "Can I get back to you tomorrow trap." Understand that people fear making a bad decision. But just as much as they fear a bad decision they fear loss. You use the fear of loss and incentives to make them want to buy today. I'll show you how to do this later.

Looking at these 4 steps, which piece do you think you are missing in your sales process?
If you are missing sales it's because you are missing one of these vital steps. NOT ONE CAN BE SKIPPED.

So let's review-

Through knowing that everything we say or do produces a feeling and a response in a person, we can therefore use certain sentences and words to predict what the person will say and how they will feel So everything I'm going to be showing you next is going to LEAD this person to want to say they NEED you, WANT you, and are excited to work with you. Through this conversation control we will also eliminate any objections.

Through the formula, conversation control, and implementing these 4 steps into our sales process we can surely make a sale. Now the question comes, how do we do this? Outlined in the next chapter is the 5 step sales process you must follow in order to increase the likelihood of making a sale.

5 Step Sales Process

Now the question comes, how do we get each of the 4 things needed to make a sale (need, emotions, value, urgency) into our sales process?

We do it by following the 5 step sales process to tie people down, get them committed and sell personal training. The five steps are these:

1) FA (Fitness Assessment) - Goal: SAY THEY NEED YOU

2) Diagrams- Goal: SEE THEY NEED YOU

3) Work out- Goal: FEEL THEY NEED YOU

4) Price preso- Goal: TIE THEM DOWN

5) Overcoming objections

1) FA

The first step in the sales process is sitting the member down and going through a fitness assessment in which you ask a series of questions to get to know the member more.

The whole purpose of the FA is not simply to ask a bunch of questions to get to know the person. THE PURPOSE OF THE FA IS TO GET THEM TO SAY THEY NEED YOU AND TO CREATE THE EMOTIONS NEEDED TO MAKE THE SALES EASY.

Again, if the person does not say themselves that they need you out loud, you most likely will not make the sale.

In the FA we are accomplishing three things:
1) Getting them to like you and trust you.
2) Creating NEED.
3) Creating emotions.

So let's start with the first one: getting someone to like you and trust you.
Your first 5-10 minutes in the FA should be getting someone to like you and trust you. Here are 6 quick ways to get someone to like you and trust you.
1) Compliment them.
2) Be energetic.
3) Be positive.
4) Relate to them (connect with them).
5) Serve them (give before you take).

6) Get to know them.

When the member walks into the room you need to get out of whatever you are doing and greet them with a warm friendly smile. Bring them over to your desk and pull out the chair for them. During this time you should have made some kind of compliment about their hair, shoes, shirt, car they drove in etc. To continue building your connection tell them about a funny thing that happened to you last weekend and then ask them how their day or weekend went. Find common ground and relate with them.

After you've built a good connection with the person and see that they are opening up, you can then proceed into the fitness assessment. DO NOT MOVE INTO THE

FITNESS ASSESSMENT WITHOUT FIRST GETTING THEM TO LIKE YOU. If you do, they will be very reluctant with opening up to you. The reason doing this is so important is because if someone doesn't trust you, they aren't going to buy from you. Secondly, if they don't like you, they also will not buy from you. Everything you are doing needs to have a purpose behind it and move you closer to making the sale.

In the fitness assessment you are going to use this little acronym: GRIDS in order to get to know the person better as well as develop the need and emotions to help close the sale. GRIDS stands for this:

GOALS

ROUTINE

DIET

SUPPLEMENTS

The NEEDS and EMOTIONS talked about
in the last chapter are created when
talking about the persons GOALS. DO
NOT SKIP THIS SECTION. MEMORIZE
EACH SENTENCE. Watch how I use
conversation control by using the
formula. Remember every statement I
make will produce a response in the
buyer and if its done properly we can
guess the answer before they even say it.
As the formula suggest, we always lead
the conversation with a question. Here's
how it should go:

Goals:

So what would be your goals? (Lose weight)

How much would you like to lose? (10lbs)

How long have you been on this journey? (3years)

Are you feeling stuck of Plateaued? (Stuck)

See you've gotten the person to say that they are stuck or plateaued. That is absolutely key because it's needed to make a sale. If they don't need me they aren't going to buy from me. In this section I know right away if someone is most likely going to buy or not.

I then move on into talking about their routine by saying something like this- "Ok Mary, you are feeling a little stuck.

What's your current routine look like?"
Mary then explains her routine to you in which you just simply say, "ok I think I see whats going on."

Now you move into the emotional side of things and get her committed to wanting to change her life. You should say something like this- "Mary what was that moment that finally got you to get out of your house and get to the gym? Or what was that moment that finally got you to turn your car into our parking lot and into our doors?!"
Hopefully she says it's because she absolutely hates how she feels or because she has a wedding coming up or something that is truly driving her. But most the time you're going to hear a simply generic answer like- "I just want to get in shape" or "I just want to be

healthy".

Listen carefully to Mary and prod her with the "WHY TECHNIQUE".
If she says, "I just wanted to get in shape."
You say, "WHY do you want to get in shape?"
"Because I don't like the way I look"
"What do you mean by that?"

With that last question you have really moved into the heart of the person and at this point they might have a tendency to cry because it's getting so personal. After they've opened up to you, you are now going to tie them down emotionally with wanting to change their life and committing to it. Your goal is to get them absolutely certain that they want to change their life and NEED to change their life; moving them from an 8 to a 10 on commitment.

Here's what you say-

TIE THEM DOWN

"So it sounds like to me that you getting in the best shape of your life is extremely important to you…. **is that right?"**

"And since you're feeling stuck, what you need most is a game plan to show you how to get there… **is that correct**?"

Remember, make sure to end your statements with a question so that they are in agreement with you. You simply making a statement doesn't not mean they agree with you even if they shake their ahead in what seems like an agreement. Get the person to say "Yes."

KEY:

If they don't open up with you, tell them your personal story of what got you started in the gym. This will usually open them up to tell you what got them started.

DIET + SUPPLEMENTS:

The reason for these last two questions in the FA is so that you can get to know what a person is doing but mainly because you can see where they are wasting their money. If they are spending hundreds of dollars on garbage food or on supplements they don't need, it is easier for them to justify spending that money on training. DO NOT ELLUDE TO USING THAT MONEY FOR PERSONAL

TRAINING YET, just find out what they are doing.

You can also include in this section something like this-

"Did you know that the average person who followed my training program saved about $300 a month on their budget!"

//Diagrams- See They Need You

After you're done going through the FA,
you now present the diagrams to them.
The purpose of the diagrams is to give
them a game plan and show them how
they are going to reach their goals. But
the real purpose from a sales stand point
is to get them to SEE THEY NEED YOU. I
have attached a copy

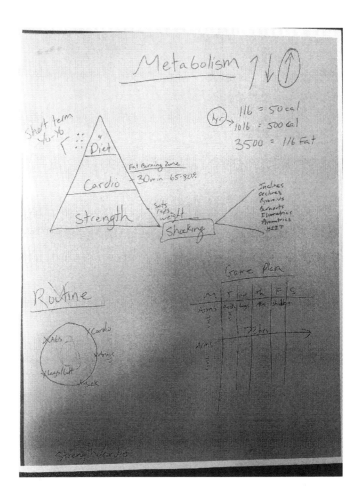

Here is the script for presenting the diagrams. As I present the programs to each potential member I am rewriting the whole thing and making it sound like if it was just for them. This is key. Remember, passion persuades. As you go through these diagrams be excited, enthusiastic and engage the member.

Let's get started-

SECTION 1: METABOLISM/MUSCLE

"Mary, it looks like we need to work with your metabolism. Have you felt that slow down at all?"

"Yeah I figured you have. Well what I want to do with you specifically is raise that back up, bring the body fat down, and for you specifically, I would like to bring your lean muscle up…here's why-

If I were to give you 1lb of lean muscle, you would burn 50 calories at rest.

A great goal for you would be 10lbs of lean muscle because you would burn 500 calories a day!

In one week thats 3,500 calories which equals 1 pound of fat! Isn't that incredible!?

Now I got to give you the bad news, it's going to take one year to gain that much lean muscle." (wait fo them to respond). "But thats ok, because you want a lifestyle change correct? Then I want you to plan on it taking a year ok?" (wait for them to respond).

"Are you sure you're ready for that kind of commitment? Great. Well I'm going to be honest with you, I need you coming to the gym 2-3x a week. Can you do that for me? Ok good."

NOTES:
As you can see, I have gotten the person to commit to a one year life change. Notice that I did not quickly brief over the one year commitment. I have challenged them and continued to challenge them with questions to make sure that they

were all in. Why did I do this? Because I can't make a 12 month program sale without them deciding for themselves that they are committing for the long haul. Secondly, I did this because the second step needed to make a sale is Emotions! This is the place where I get them bought in and committed to changing their life.

SECTION 2: PYRAMID

"Now Mary there are 3 ways to reach your goals.

You have your diet at the top. On a scale of 1-10 how good is your diet? We want to teach you 6 meals a day because this will raise your metabolism.

Secondly is your cardio. I need you to be in what's called the Fat Burning Zone. In order for you to get the most weight loss, you need to be in this zone. It's 30 min with a heart rate between 65-80%. In other words when you walk through the doors and get on a tread mill, you basically need to hold a jog pace for 30 min. Your heart should be beating strong and you should start feeling sweat come down your forehead.

Now these two pieces are what I like to call the SHORT TERM. Meaning you can lose a good amount of weight from those two alone, but the problem with them is that they are a Yo-Yo. As soon as you stop you are going right back where you were before. Now I got to imagine Mary that you are a lot like me. There are days when I am gone on vacation or have parties to attend to; or there are days where I have just exhausted myself at work and the last thing I want to do is get into the gym and work out. And the last thing I want to see happen is you go back to where you were before and waste all that time.

That is why I don't want you focusing on those two alone and why you should focus on this last piece of the diagram called strength. The reason for this is because even when you're not in the gym your muscle is still burning calories.

You will have a certain amount of sets, reps and weight that you should be following. But you can do this 7 days a week and still get no results. Thats why the most important thing that you need to do is called shocking your muscle. Have you ever heard that term before?

Basically you need to continually change up your work outs all the time in order to continue seeing results. How do we change up your work outs? By doing

inclines, declines, pyramids, burnouts, isometrics, plyometrics and burnouts. Have you ever heard of these before? You haven't?
Ok great, well I am going to have fun teaching you them all."

NOTES:
The key to this section is getting them to say that they have never done the different types of shocking muscles you have listed. This gets them to SEE that they NEED you. You just told them that the only way they can get results is by shocking their muscles and when you ask them if they've done it before they are admitting that they cant do it on their own and therefore need you to teach them.
If you do not show this section you will constantly get people at the end of your

presentation saying to you that they want to try it on their own. The only reason why someone would say that they want to do it on their own instead of using a trainer is because they don't feel like they need you. People truly think they know how to continually change up their workouts but the reality is they don't and this section SHOWS them that.

SECTION 3: ROUTINE/GAMEPLAN

Mary, the worst thing you could possibly do is a routine. And this is what I did when I first started at the gym. Basically I would come in and do my cardio and then after that I would bounce around to the different machines. I would hit my arms, then move to my back, then legs, and finally I would hit my abs. This was my Monday, Wednesday, and Friday work out. And just like me, I promise that 3 months from now you won't see any changes.

Here's what you need to do….here's your game plan:

On Monday you are just going to do your arms. Instead of doing just one or two machines you're going to do about four, five, or six different work outs; hitting all the different angles. Then you'll move to your back where once again you'll do multiple different work outs. Then shoulders, abs and so forth.

Now here is the key Mary….when you get back to week two you're going to hit the arms again but it's a totally different work out. That's what I mean by shocking your muscles. Here's why, you've torn down the muscle and it's gotten bigger, better, and stronger. Therefore its going to need a bigger, better, and stronger work out if you expect to see improvement. Does that make sense?

And we waited a week because it takes 72 hours for your muscle to repair. That's also why we can't hit them right away. Now what you specifically need is what's called a strength cardio workout. One in which we get your heart rate up so we are burning weight that way as well as building the muscle up and burning weight that way also.

NOTES:

Notice that I never want to make the potential client feel ashamed and will therefore relate to them by saying, "And this is what I did when I started."

You see the beautiful thing about these diagrams is that the client knows exactly what they need to do in order to reach their goals and at the same time they have no clue how to implement it. It's a double edge sword that gets them to need you more and commits them to a 12 month program. The diagrams are one aspect in the sales process that you never want to skip. This sheet of paper also gives them a game plan that they get to keep which was one of the incentives. At the end of explaining this, they should be completely blown away.

//Work Out: Feel They Need You

The workout should be the icing on the cake in your selling presentation. You have just gotten the client committed to changing their life and gotten them all excited about changing their life; you got them to say they were stuck which made them verbally say they need you and finally through the diagrams you showed them they need you. Now your final step before the price presentation is to get them to FEEL they need you.

Your work out should be UNIQUE, FUN, INTERESTING, AND SHOW THEM WHY HAVING A TRAINER IS THE BEST DECISION IN THE WORLD.

Everyone buys a trainer for different

reasons. Your work out should encompass the 4 areas that people lose over the course of time: strength, endurance, balance, and range of motion. I can't tell you how many times I have sold a training program simply because the person had no balance or because their range of motion was half of what it should be.

Touching on each of those four areas is crucial because I've worked with dozens of people who told me straight up they weren't buying personal training and only wanted the free session, but afterwards ended up buying training because they never realized how bad they were in balance or range of motion. And since they don't know how to do balance workouts or increase their range of motion, they would end up buying. These clients need to understand that unless they start implementing those 4 things into their current routine they are going to have some serious problems in 5 to 10 years from where they are. It's imperative that you be honest with them. Nobody wants a raised toilet seat because they have no range of motion in their legs and can't sit down anymore. Nobody wants a cane or walker simply because they never did balance workouts.

Most people don't realize how bad their balance and range of motion is. I mean seriously, when is the last time you've seen a 45yr old man tell his wife that he is going to do a random balance test on himself?

Your work outs should never touch a machine. If they use machines, why on earth would they need you? Get them to understand that there are multiple pieces to every muscle (the shoulder has 3 muscles to it, the bicep has two angles to it, the tricep has three muscles to it etc.) and that a machine will only usually work one of those angles. Explain to them that a trainer doesn't usually use a machine because it can't get their heart rate up and also doesn't hit all the angles to every muscle.

With these simple tools you can create a work out that gets them to feel that they need you.

//Price Presentation

The biggest obstacle I have ever seen in selling personal training is how to transition from the work out to the prices without it sounding abrupt. Here is a simple little script to follow in order to alleviate yourself from that-

Did you have fun today?
Did you like the work out?
Did you learn something new?
(These three sentences are here because they get your client in the YES mode. It seems stupid but honestly it really works. Your mind is very interesting. It focus' on rhythms and patterns and responds because of it. Here is an example. Try and

answer this questions before reading the answer. If I am 4 years old and my brother is half my age, how old is he by the time I'm 40? If you answered 20, you are wrong. Let's change the wording so your brain can find the answer faster. If I am 4 years old and my brother is two years younger (half my age), how old is he when I am 40? Obviously the answer is now 38. You see your brain picked up on the word HALF YOUR AGE and came to a quick conclusion. That's what these 3 little sentences are doing. Let's continue on).

You did awesome today! Seriously I was really proud of everything you did.
(Why is this sentence here? Remember your words create feelings and we want the client to like you more and trust you more. These words are here to build your

rapport. The second phrase that starts with the word "seriously" is there because you want them to know that your not just flattering them, but are serious about what you are saying).

After observing everything today, I FEEL like you have the passion, commitment, and energy to reaching your goal. I feel like the only thing you are missing is the knowledge of all the different work outs... would you agree?

Seriously, apart from that what would you possibly be missing?!

Someone with your same goals will usually see a trainer 2-3x a week. But obviously money is a concern for everyone, so let's find a program that fits your needs and budget ok?

Great.

(Ok, there is a LOT going on in this paragraph. Notice first that I am saying, "after observing everything today," in other words I have been watching everything that has been happening and therefore have something to share. The next words are "I FEEL." These words are absolutely crucial for you. You are NOT telling them that they are missing knowledge of all the different work outs as if to put them in a defense mode. You are saying you FEEL like they are missing knowledge of the different work outs. In other words you're taking a humble approach knowing that you could be wrong. And the sentence ends with, "would you agree?" to get a mutual understanding and reaffirming to the client again that without you they can't do

it on their own. They need you because they lack the knowledge of the work outs. Notice the beauty of the last sentence?! Basically you got them to agree to buying training as long as it fit in their needs and budget. Thats your goal! Find a program that works for them and they are ready to buy. You basically made the sale right there).

We have two different programs we offer. We have a 6 month program and a 12 month program. The only difference between the two is the price per session. The 6 month is $65 a session and the 12 month is $55 a session. The more you get the cheaper it gets. Based on your goals and what you're looking to accomplish I would recommend the 12 month program but which one are you most interested in and I'll explain further.

(Notice that you are presenting the programs and then recommending one to them. The very last sentence is extremely important. You are narrowing down the programs to be able to explain further how the programs work. A common error I see with trainers and presenting programs is that they show them all and say, "well what do you think?"

To which the client will respond, "I need to think about it." And you have no clue where to go from there. I mean what are they thinking about? The length of the program or how many sessions? Or maybe its how much they want to spend? You don't know because you haven't narrowed down the programs. It's like taking a loved one to a restaurant with a giant menu. In order to help them decide the waitress will help narrow down the menu by saying, "Are you interested in chicken, lasagna, or salads?" By narrowing down the waitress can now explain further what they have.)

Great. In the 12 month program you have three different options. You can work with a trainer 1x a week, 2x a week, or 3x a week.

Our 1x a week program we like to call it the "Do It On Your Own Program." This is where you would meet your trainer on Monday and then your trainer would write you homework assignments for Wednesday and Friday.

Our most popular option is the 2x a week program. That's where you would see your trainer on Monday, then on Wednesday you would get your homework assignment and then you would see your trainer again on Friday.

Last but not least is our 3x a week program where you see your trainer every single time you come to the gym. Obviously the more you see a trainer the better the results you're going to get. **Of these programs which one would you like to get started with today?**

(Notice in the last sentence I am using an assumptive close. I am not asking what they think or if they want to do it. I am assuming they want to train because they have admitted over and over that they need it and want to change their life.)

// **OVERCOMING OBJECTIONS**

At this point in the presentation the client will say either one of three things-
I want to think about it
I need to talk to my spouse
I don't have the money

At this point it doesn't matter what they say. You will use conversation control and lead the person where they need to go. It is imperative that you have a belief that everyone you sit with wants a trainer. I mean think about it this way, if training was free wouldn't everyone want to do it? So with this belief know that there are no excuses besides money. It always comes down to the money and it's your job to lead them into a program that fits their needs and budget.

As soon as they say an objection you're going to say-
"I totally understand….which one are you leaning towards?"

At this point 95% of the time they will say the 1x a week and you should respond with-
"Did you like the program today? Can you see yourself doing it in the future? Is what you're feeling is that $220 is a little outside the budget?"

At this point they are going to say, "yes."

From here you want to say,
"Well I might be able to give you my employee discount. Would that help you out at all?"

They will respond, "Possibly. What's it drop it to?"

Say, "It will drop it down to $200 a month. Is that better for you?"

One out of 6 people will actually think that is a great deal and buy from you. The other 5 will say, "I appreciate it, but I need to go home and think about it."

At this point you need to keep the conversation going and lead them once again with these words-

"Unfortunately that's all I can do. But what if I got permission to customize a program for you? Instead of doing 4x a month, what if we just met 2 or 3x a month? I can still get you nutritional guidance and write up a plan for you on the days you're not with me. Would that be better? Great. How many sessions would you like me to see that I can approve?

Now you got the sale!!!

KEY TO CLOSING:

Get the client to unfold a number. Once you know what they can afford on a monthly basis you can immediately come up with a game plan on how to help them. Unless they say a number, you can't help them.

Remember people don't want to feel like they are being sold. They want to leave their interaction with you feeling like they got a good deal or that you helped them out.

Also notice this, I am not selling handfuls of sessions like most trainers do. I want monthly EFT and I also want them committed to a program of 6 months of 12 months. I now have a steady income that keeps growing over time and I wont be burning through clients since they are committing to a long time frame.

If you did want to sell handfuls of sessions and still follow these scripts, then I would suggest offering 24, 48, and 96 sessions only and following the scripts from there.

Conversation Control Price Press
Script 2

WHICH ONE WOULD YOU LIKE TO GET
STARTED WITH TODAY?

— — — — — — —->

I NEED TO THINK ABOUT IT

TOTALLY UNDERSTAND….WHICH
ONE ARE YOU LEANING TOWARDS?

— — — —>

4X A MONTH

DID YOU LIKE THE PROGRAM TODAY?
CAN YOU SEE YOURSELF DOING IT
IN THE FUTURE?
IS WHAT YOU'RE FEELING IS THAT ITS

A LITTLE OUTSIDE THE BUDGET?

————————>

YES

I MIGHT BE ABLE TO GIVE YOU MY
EMPLOYEE DISCOUNT. WOULD THAT
HELP?

——————————->

POSSIBLY. WHAT IS IT?

IT WOULD BRING IT TO
$200 A MONTH. IS THAT BETTER?

————————————>

NO. I NEED TO THINK ABOUT IT.

UNFORTUNATLY THATS ALL I CAN DO.
HOW CLOSE TO $200 CAN YOU GET
TO?
WOULD 190 WORK?

180?

170?

$————————> IF

IT WAS MORE LIKE $150

SO WHAT YOUR TELLING ME IS THAT
IF THERE WAS A PROGRAM AROUND
150 THAT WOULD BE MORE
COMFORTABLE?

$————————->

YES.

OK LET ME GO SEE WHAT I CAN DO.

SALE MADE!!!!

CONVERSATION CONTROL PRICE PRESO SCRIPT 3

WHICH ONE WOULD YOU LIKE TO GET
STARTED WITH TODAY?

$$— — — — — — —->$$

I NEED TO THINK ABOUT IT

TOTALLY UNDERSTAND….WHICH
ONE ARE YOU LEANING TOWARDS?

$$— — — —>$$

4X A MONTH

DID YOU LIKE THE PROGRAM TODAY?
CAN YOU SEE YOURSELF DOING IT
IN THE FUTURE?
IS WHAT YOUR FEELING IS THAT ITS

A LITTLE OUTSIDE THE BUDGET?

─ ─ ─ ─ ─ ─ ─>

YES

I MIGHT BE ABLE TO GIVE YOU MY
EMPLOYEE DISCOUNT. WOULD THAT
HELP?

─ ─ ─ ─ ─ ─ ─ ─ ─>

POSSIBLY. WHAT IS IT?

IT WOULD BRING IT TO
$200 A MONTH. IS THAT BETTER?

─ ─ ─ ─ ─ ─ ─ ─ ─ ─>

NO. I NEED TO THINK ABOUT IT.

UNFORTUNATLY THAT'S ALL I CAN DO.
ON A POSITIVE NOTE WE HAVE
COUPONS

HAPPENING ALL THE TIME THAT
SOMETIMES
DROP IT MORE THAT WHAT I CAN DO.
WOULD
YOU LIKE ME TO CALL YOU IF I GOT
ONE?

————————>

YES!

GREAT! NOW I DON'T WANT TO
BOMBARD YOU
WITH A MILLION PHONE CALLS.
WHAT'S A
GENERAL PRICE YOU WANTED TO BE
AROUND
AND I'LL CALL YOU WHEN WE HAVE
SOMETHING
AROUND THAT.

————————> $150

THE ONLY THING I CAN THINK OF TO
HELP YOU

IS THAT WE HAD A COUPON FROM A
COUPLE

WEEKS PAST. I DON'T KNOW IF IT'S
STILL

AVAILABLE AND HONESTLY I DONT
KNOW

IF IT WENT THAT LOW. BUT WOULD
YOU

LIKE ME TO ASK MY BOSS?

—————> YEA!

CONVERSATION CONTROL PRICE PRESO 4: BUDGET CLOSE SCRIPT

This script only works for those who are about 28years old and younger and should only be used once a solid rapport has been developed.

The key is that while you are in the middle of the work out you are going to drop a hint at them letting them know that training is expensive. They will say, "Yea I figured it was expensive." Follow up with, "When we get back to the desk I want to try and help you."

This will create excitement in their heart and make them feel appreciative of you for helping them out.

At the desk you want to say, "Like I said, training can be expensive and I don't want you paying for something that is outside your budget but I got some ideas on how to help you. Lets go over your budget to figure out how much you can afford on a monthly basis."

At this point ask them how much money they make a month. (Now I think you understand why you cant ask that question to someone over 28.)

After finding out how much money they make ask them what their expenses are (car payment, rent, etc). Whatever money is left over you want to ask them, "How much of this money left over would you like to invest towards training and I can see what program I can come up with."

At this point you have the sale!

How much do you make a month?

$-------->$

$1,200

What are your expenses?

$------->$ $200

for car, $50 for credit card.

You have about $950 left
over...how much would you
like to put toward training?

$-------->$

$360 I can do.

Ok, let me go see what I can do.

After the sale is made, let them know that you don't want them sharing the deal you gave them with anyone else. This will make them feel special and leave feeling like you really helped them out. Also, get them willing to write a review for you.

//MORE CLOSING TECHNIQUES

The reason why most people can't close training sales is because they run out of ammo with what to say next. They key is keeping the conversation going and making the person feel like you are trying to help them and understand their situation.

If you don't feel like you can memorize the scripts above, a real simple formula to remember when overcoming an objection is-

SYMPATHIZE

REPEAT

RELATE

ISOLATE

Here's how it works:

When someone says that they need to talk to their spouse you are going to say-

SYMPATHIZE- "I totally understand you want....

REPEAT- "that you want to talk with your spouse

RELATE- "in fact whenever I make important decisions I usually like to talk it over also"

ISOLATE- "Let me ask you, when you go home to talk with your spouse....are you going to talk to them about wanting to get in shape or would it be a bout the money?"

Obviously they are going to say it's about the money. From here keep the conversation going by saying something like, So do you think they will be excited for you and glad that you want to do training, or do you feel that they are probably going to shut you down because its to much money?"

"Yea, so it sounds like to me that this 4x a month program doesn't quite fit into your budget right now. Is that correct? Well I would imagine you have a good idea of what your budget is and what would be comfortable with your spouse....if you were to pick a number between $50/month and $200, what do you think would be best?"

This works for any objection-

Think about it

"I totally understand you want to think about it. In fact I always like to process everything as well. When you go home to think about it, are you mainly going to think about getting in the best shape of your life or more about the money?"

Time

"I totally understand that time is very tight for you. In fact, I struggle with the very same thing myself. But let me ask you, if I were to make it so you had total flexibility with your scheduling of your sessions and allowed all your sessions to roll over so that you never lose them, is there anything else that would keep you from getting started with me?"

How To Close With Faster

Here is what you do when you've followed all the steps, but still can't seem to get them committed to a program and they say things like, "I don't know what my budget is or if I can afford it"

"So you already said you liked the program and you can see yourself doing this correct?... What it sounds like to me is that you're thinking-
"I have this expense, this payment, and this cost" and you're not even sure that you can fit training into your budget, does that sound right?
Yea that's what I thought you were thinking, in fact a lot of people who look to

begin a program feel the same way. I want you to know that it's not your budget that pays for training, but your expenses.

Let me ask you, would you agree that there are certain things in your life that need to be changed in order for you to get to where you're trying to go?
I'm glad you agree.
And honestly, I need you to know that if you're desiring to work with me I NEED YOU to change those things. Are you willing to do that?

Now when I began this same journey you're on, here's what I found out-
That through my expenses I was spending over $500 a month on things that were keeping me from my goals. Isn't that crazy? The average American

spends about $360 a month on random stuff that keeps them from their goals. Where would you say you're at?

NOW CHECK THIS OUT:
Show picture of meal prep food.
How much do you think this costs?
Literally like $15.
You're saving so much money.

Grab your phone for me really quick, I got homework for you.

HERES YOUR HOMEWORK:
1) Go to your local grocery story and buy a bag of chicken, broccoli and yogurt.
2) Get your resting heart rate. I'm going to need that tomorrow to calculate your THR to make sure we will get the progress we

need. You're going to have specific numbers you need to be at.

3) Download My Fitness Pal. For the next two weeks I need you to keep track of everything you're eating.

MONEY:

How much of the $360 would you be willing to invest into you're training? Remember I need you to eventually get rid of this all.

The reason you are having them look at a photo, having them grab their phone, and giving them homework assignments, is because you are assuming the sale and getting them excited about starting their journey. This will make the sales process smoother and easier. It shows confidence.

//SUMMARY

This is the process you need to follow if you want the most success in selling big training packages.

Get them to NEED you...

Get them EMOTIONALLY excited and committed...

Get them to see how awesome it is working with you....

Give them a reason to buy today and not tomorrow....

Lead the conversations with questions. Be genuine, excited, sincere.

And most of all KNOW at the end of the

day…

 YOU ARE IN CONTROL…

…of how they FEEL ….and how they RESPOND.

It's all based on your presentation.

Lead well and you will do well.

You'll surely get somewhere….the question is where.

//Floor Pull Scripts

The key to pulling someone off the floor and into an assessment is making sure they don't feel like they are being singled out. There must be a REASON on why you are approaching them otherwise they will push you away and say no. Here is a list of 6 ways I have used to generate personal training leads.

1)You have a one on one training session on your account….when are you coming into the gym next?

2) Hey mam/sir…I'm one of the managers here. When you came in your account set

me an alert….you have a huge discount off of your training…did anyone ever tell you?

The reason I stopped you was because it was about to expire. Have you ever thought of working with a trainer before? Cool, let's go back to the desk and I can show you your options.

3) Hey mam/sir…I'm one of the managers here. When you came in your account set me an alert….you had a one on one training session on your account that was about to expire…when are you coming into the gym next?
As long as it is scheduled you will not lose it.

4) Cleaning Approach:
When you see someone cleaning up the

gym go up to them and say this-
"Thank you so much for cleaning up the gym. I've been trying to make this place look more clean and I really appreciate you taking care of everything. Because of your help, I'm going to give you a $100 training session for free. When are you coming into the gym next?"

5) Turning a Complaint Into An Assessment
"I'm so sorry about _____. I'll make sure to get that fixed right away. Because of your inconvenience I'm going to give you a $100 training session. When are you coming into the gym next?"

6) Member Appreciation Day
"Hey_____, for member appreciation day we are giving away one on one training

sessions. When are you coming into the gym next?"

7) Hey_____, my name is Mike. "I'm one of the trainers here and I've worked out with almost every single person to make sure they have a game plan for success. I don't think I've ever had the privilege to work with you…how long have you been here for?
(keep small conversation going focused on them. Always ask questions.)
Eventually end with, "So when are you coming into the gym next?"

8) Another great way to get leads is to take a sheet of paper with a list of times available….go around to everyone in the gym and say, "For member appreciation day we are giving away free training

sessions…when would you like to use yours?"

Then show them the time slots and have them put their name and number in it.

You can also leave that sheet of paper at the front desk with a sign next to it saying that all new members receive a free training session.

Phone Scripts

"Hey _____, this is _____ with ___(your gym)_____. I just wanted to welcome you to the club. I'm one of the managers here and when you joined you were given a one on one training session and I just wanted to schedule that for you. When is the next time you're coming to the gym?"

If they say, "Can I get back to you?" say back, "Well the reason why I am calling is because your session is about to expire. As long as it's in the system you won't lose it. Is there a day that works better for you?"

Made in the
USA
Columbia, SC